MW01094539

Hemorrhoids No More

The Complete Guide On Hemorrhoids
Causes & Symptoms, Hemorrhoids
Treatments, & How Never To Have
Hemorrhoids Ever Again!

Thomas Barrett

Hemorrhoids No More

Publisher: Living Plus Healthy Publishing

ISBN-13: 978-1499316582

ISBN-10: 1499316585

Disclaimer

The Publisher has strived to be as accurate and complete as possible in the creation of this book. While all attempts have been made to verify information provided in this publication, the Publisher assumes no responsibility for errors, omissions, or contrary interpretation of the subject matter herein. Any perceived slights of specific persons, peoples, or organizations are unintentional.

This book is not intended for use as a source of legal, business, accounting or financial advice. All readers are advised to seek services of competent professionals in the legal, business, accounting, and finance fields.

The information in this book is not intended or implied to be a substitute for professional medical advice, diagnosis or treatment. All content contained in this book is for general information purposes only. Always consult your healthcare provider before carrying on any health program.

Table of Contents

Introduction

There are few gastrointestinal problems that people talk about less than hemorrhoids. They are a forbidden item of discussion among friends, even family members. And yet they can be extremely uncomfortable and, in many cases, treatable only by doctors who are experts in handling these little annoyances.

Are you among those who suffer from hemorrhoids? Statistics show that 50 percent of American adults have hemorrhoids by the age of 50. Only a very small percent of these people actually attempt to seek treatment for their condition. This amounts to about 10.4 million people in the US having hemorrhoids and seeking treatment. In addition, each year an additional 1 million new cases among Americans develop. About 10-20 percent of all cases eventually need surgery.

Not everyone has symptoms from their hemorrhoids but 23 million people in the US or about 12.8 percent of adults have internal hemorrhoids and are symptomatic. About 1.9 million people receive treatment as outpatients for their condition in ambulatory care units. For people older than 45 years of age, 25 percent of sufferers are women and 15 percent of sufferers are men. This is because women tend to get hemorrhoids in pregnancy and once they get them, they tend not to go away.

Some people have a genetic predisposition that makes them more likely to get hemorrhoids. If you have several family members who have hemorrhoids, you should practice good hygiene and do what you can to avoid getting hemorrhoids. Yes, they are preventable.

The risk of getting hemorrhoids goes up with age and it is unlikely you'll get the condition before age 30 unless you have them from pregnancy. The main reasons people get hemorrhoids are straining at stool, constipation, heavy lifting and pregnancy.

As you'll read about in the next few chapters, hemorrhoids are nothing more than dilated anal veins. Just as you have veins in the rest of your body, there is a plexus or ring of veins around the anus. And being veins, they are very elastic and stretch when pressure is put upon them. Pressure can come from constipation or the weight of a fetal head on the anus in the later stages of pregnancy.

If enough pressure is put on the anal veins for long enough period of time, the veins begin to stretch out and dilate, forming what appears to be lumps on the outside of the anus. Alternatively, your hemorrhoids can be on the inside of your anus and may not be visible or palpable from the outside. In either case, the veins are dilated and more delicate than if the veins were completely normal. Being delicate, they tend to bleed, even with wiping oneself or having a hard stool.

As you'll see in the rest of this book, hemorrhoids can be annoying but they aren't dangerous. With judicious treatment and sometimes medical help, you should be able to live with condition.

Chapter 1: What Are Hemorrhoids?

As you learned in the introduction, hemorrhoids are nothing more than dilated, spongy veins that can be on the outside of the anus or inside the anus, where they can't be seen. On the outside, they feel like soft lumps unless a blood clot forms in the lump and it becomes a hard, painful lump. Let's take a look at the anatomy of the anus and the anatomy of hemorrhoids.

Hemorrhoids are cushions of vascular tissue that are basically normal-sized in most people. The hemorrhoids drain blood away from the anal area, which is considered a highly vascular area. Inside the anal canal are three primary cushions, located in the left lateral anus, the right anterior anus and the right posterior anus. In a sense, they form a ring.

These hemorrhoidal cushions do not bother people unless they become damaged or diseased in some way. These cushions technically aren't arteries and they aren't veins. Instead they are special sets of blood vessels known as sinusoids, consisting of smooth muscle, connective tissue and blood. This collection of blood vessels is called the hemorrhoidal plexus. They are very vascular and bleed a lot when nicked or cut.

The hemorrhoidal plexus is important for stool continence. It is believed that these cushions contribute to up to twenty percent of the pressure of anal closure and protect the anal sphincter muscles as stool passes the anus. You get symptoms of hemorrhoids when the hemorrhoidal cushions slide down from their original position and end up partly outside the body. You also get symptoms when the pressure in the venous system of the anus is increased, feeding back that increase in pressure to the sinusoids.

There are two types of hemorrhoids: the internal hemorrhoids which arise from the superior hemorrhoidal plexus and the external hemorrhoids from the inferior hemorrhoidal plexus. There is a line called the dentate line that separates the interior from the exterior hemorrhoidal plexuses.

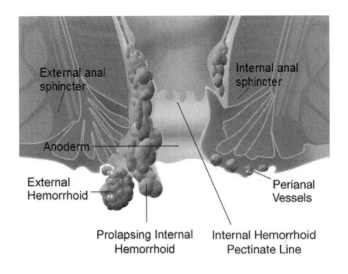

External anal sphincter

Internal anal sphincter

Anoderm

External Hemorrhoid

Perianal Vessels

Prolapsing Internal Hemorrhoid

Internal Hemorrhoid Pectinate Line

Internal Hemorrhoids

You can't see or feel internal hemorrhoids as they lie inside the rectum about a fingers length from view. Because they are not covered with skin, they do not generally hurt, even when inflamed and swollen. Generally, bleeding is the only symptom you get when the internal hemorrhoids have become engorged; however, these hemorrhoids can stretch downward and can prolapse through the anus, causing increased bleeding and the feeling of a large lump coming through the anus. Prolapsed hemorrhoids can actually hurt but, fortunately they recede back into the rectum on their own so that no medical attention is needed. You or your doctor can also push them into place without difficulty.

Internal hemorrhoids can be completely asymptomatic until you have a bowel movement. Then the stool rubs against the hemorrhoids, causing them to bleed, often profusely. The stool will be bloody, usually on the outside of the stool.

Internal hemorrhoids are not covered by skin but by columnar epithelium, the same tissue that covers the inside of the rectum. There are no pain fibers in columnar epithelium. Internal hemorrhoids can be classified or graded as to the amount of prolapse the hemorrhoid has. For example:

- Grade I hemorrhoid—does not prolapse and is merely a prominent blood vessel

- Grade II hemorrhoid—this prolapses when you bear down but suck back in spontaneously when you are not straining.

- Grade III hemorrhoid—this prolapses upon bearing down and needs manual reduction.

- Grade IV hemorrhoid—the hemorrhoid is prolapsed and cannot be manually reduced.

Fortunately, even high grade hemorrhoids can be treated with surgical treatment. This will be discussed in a later chapter.

External Hemorrhoids

External hemorrhoids are covered with skin so they can become irritated or painful. They feel like grape-sized or smaller lumps around the anus. Generally they are just irritating to have and don't hurt unless stool collects around them, causing itching and burning of the hemorrhoids. External hemorrhoids can become clotted with dried blood forming a larger grape-sized painful and purple hard lump. This often needs to be treated under the care of a doctor and they can become extremely uncomfortable.

A Warning

The main symptom of hemorrhoids, both internal and external is bleeding. If you experience bleeding from the anus, with or without a bowel movement, you need to know that there are far more serious things that can cause the same kind of bleeding.

The worst is colorectal cancer, which can cause a change in bowel movements, weight loss and bleeding from the anus, usually with a bowel movement. Just because you have hemorrhoids doesn't mean that the hemorrhoids are the cause of the bleeding. If you have a strong family history of colorectal cancer or are over the age of 50 years, you need to strongly consider having a screening colonoscopy for colon polyps or colon cancer. This can be a lifesaving preventative examination that you should have if you are a candidate for the test. Never assume it is hemorrhoids as that can be a deadly decision.

Differential Diagnosis

The differential diagnosis involves a list of other things could be wrong when it seems like a hemorrhoid. For example, a hemorrhoid could instead be a rectal fissure, a rectal fistula, a skin tag, abscesses (collections of infection) or, as noted above, colorectal cancer. Besides colon cancer, inflammatory bowel disease, diverticular disease and other colonic diseases can bleed painlessly. There is a condition called anorectal varices which are swollen veins caused by liver disease or other cause of portal hypertension. They can feel like hemorrhoids but, in fact, they are not.

Summary

Hemorrhoids are common and annoying swollen areas of the hemorrhoidal cushions. There are hemorrhoidal cushions above and below the dentate line, leading to "internal" and "external" hemorrhoids. The main symptom of the disease is rectal bleeding. Depending on the location of the hemorrhoids and their size, they may be painful or may not be painful. It's important to remember that serious diseases can also mimic hemorrhoids so that if you have rectal bleeding and are of the risk category for colorectal cancer, you need to see a doctor.

Chapter 2: The One Product That Saved My Life

I placed this chapter here for those who are reading this book and in need of a fast, immediate solution to their hemorrhoids problems.

I know how you feel because I was in your shoes before. I want to share with you the one product that has worked for me. However, remember that this or any other hemorrhoids treatments can only reduce symptoms temporarily. To be permanently free from hemorrhoids you need to read the rest of this book and undergo lifestyle changes it suggests.

First, the disclaimer: I am not affiliated with the product manufacture and I do not get paid for recommending this product. I cannot guarantee that you will get the same result as I. I can only tell you my personal experience as is.

In 2001 I had a severe external hemorrhoids outbreak. It turned very bad within 2 days. The piles were huge. I had lots of bleeding and excruciating pain every time I had a bowel movement.

I wasn't able to sit, walk, stand, or even sleep. I tried every over the counter medicine and methods suggested over the Internet but only to get very brief relief. I was too embarrassed to go to the doctor and hoped that it would just go away. But it just got worse and worse as time went on.

After 2 weeks I just couldn't take it anymore and was ready to see a doctor. But I thought I would search the Internet one last time. A product called "PILEX" (not to be confused with "Himalaya Pilex" which is a totally different product) jumped out at me. I was intrigued by the testimonials where many people claimed how fast and how well it worked.

There are two options for PILEX. The basic one is for mild hemorrhoids relief. It only has 7 capsules in the bottle. Yes, only 7. You take them once a day orally for 7 days. That's it. It claims your hemorrhoids will be gone by the end of 7 days.

The second option, PILEX Max, is for chronic or long term hemorrhoidal conditions. It has 14 capsules for one-week supply. You take 2 capsules a day for 7 days.

PILEX is not cheap. In fact, it's very expensive. The basic option is $37 – that's over $5 per capsule. PILEX Max is $57, or over $4 per capsule.

However, I was so desperate that I would try anything. I would gladly pay $57; heck, I would be willing to pay $5,700 if I could just get rid of those hemorrhoids!

There was no question that I needed the PILEX Max. I ordered from the manufacture's web site (www.pilex.com) with express shipping and got it the next day.

I started to take two capsules in the morning as directed. Nothing happened on the first day. But on the second day the pain lessened and it turned into somewhat a numb feeling. The piles, however, were about the same size.

On the third day the pain was greatly reduced. The bleeding stopped and the piles started to shrink.

Fourth day – no more pain! The piles continued to shrink. On the fifth day the hemorrhoids were almost gone. Actually, it was reduced to a very small bump but never completely disappears. However, it is no longer painful.

I continued to take the remaining capsules until the 7th day. The web site says once you finish the bottle you will be hemorrhoid-free for at least 6 months.

I ordered a second bottle right away. That experience was so painful that I would not take any chances. I wanted to have a bottle at hand just in case.

I also began to exercise more and ate more fiber-rich food. Things were going well until 2007 when I went to a 4-day business conference in Chicago. I was not eating well and had a bad constipation on the 3rd day. Then the hemorrhoids came back.

I was horrified. I had been hemorrhoid-free for so many years that I forgot to pack PILEX with me. I left the conference half day early in fear of the outbreak. Fortunately, when I got home the piles had just begun to enlarge. I had pain and some bleeding but not as serious as the last time.

I took PILEX right away and all the symptoms were gone in 2 days. I have not had any outbreak since. Never will I leave home without PILEX ever again!

As mentioned before, only lifestyle and diet changes will give you long term results. But that takes time and if you are in excruciating pain now, you want it gone right now. Not tomorrow, not next week. NOW! You may want to give PILEX Max a try. Like I said, I can't guarantee it will work for you but I can tell you it did save my life.

Chapter 3: What Causes Hemorrhoids?

Anything that increases the pressure of the rectal vasculature—the veins in particular—can result in hemorrhoids. How all this works is not completely clear but doctors have found that a lack of exercise triggers hemorrhoids. In addition, constipation or diarrhea (a change in bowel habits) can cause irritation of the veins around the anus.

People who have ascites, which is an increase in abdominal fluid pressure, usually from liver disease, can get hemorrhoids as can people who eat low fiber diets. Prolonged straining at stool can result in hemorrhoids. Pregnancy results in a fetal head increasing the anal pressure and resultant hemorrhoids. Genetics can play a role, such as being born with an absence of valves inside the hemorrhoidal veins. People who sit too much at their job can get hemorrhoids as a result. People who are obese can get hemorrhoids.

Also during pregnancy, hormones can change and can cause the hemorrhoidal vessels to enlarge, even if the fetus is small and isn't putting pressure on the anal veins. Unfortunately, during delivery, the fetus really increases the pressure on the anal veins and hemorrhoids that weren't there just before the delivery. Many of the hemorrhoids pass after the delivery, although some don't.

In summary, the main reasons you can get hemorrhoids are:

- Straining at stooling
- Sitting a long time, especially on the toilet
- Genetic defects
- Chronic diarrhea
- Chronic constipation
- Obesity
- Pregnancy
- Anal intercourse
- Older age
- Ascites of the liver

How Can You Prevent Hemorrhoids?

Now that you know the causes of hemorrhoids, you can see where there might be some things you can do to prevent them. The trouble with hemorrhoids is that, once you get them, they tend not to go away on their own. If hemorrhoids run in your family or if you feel as though hemorrhoids are coming on, go straight to prevention so they won't get serious.

The first thing you should do is **avoid becoming constipated whenever possible**. This means including high fiber foods in your diet such as fruits, whole vegetables, beans, and whole grains. Change your diet to include whole grain bread instead of white bread, which is highly processed and can contribute to constipation. Drink plenty of fluids, at least 10-12 glasses of water per day. It not only protects your urinary system but your bowels are protected from having constipated stools.

Get a little bit of exercise each day for about 2 1/2 hours per week if it's moderate exercise. If what you can do is vigorous exercise, you can get that down to half that or 1 1/4 hours per week. It doesn't have to be a big chunk of activity. Just get ten minutes of activity at a time, three times a day throughout the day.

If these natural tips and trick don't relieve your constipation, take an over the counter fiber supplement such as Metamucil or Citrucel. Take it as directed once daily, starting with smaller doses and increasing gradually until you find a dose that works for you and keeps you regular. Try to have a bowel movement at the same time of the day. If you stick to a regular routine, you'll strain less. Take your time with a bowel movement so that you don't strain. Let your colon do all the work for you so you don't have to push as hard.

Make sure you go to the bathroom as soon as you have the urge and then just let things happen completely naturally. If you're holding your breath during a bowel movement, that's too much pressure on the anal veins. Don't read on the toilet as that can trigger you to sit there longer. As soon as your bowel movement is done, get off the toilet.

It's surprising how much your daily activities affect your bowels. If you work at an office desk, get up frequently for walking breaks and try not to lift heavy objects too much. Exhale as you are lifting heavy objects; if you are holding your breath, you are straining and putting too much abdominal pressure on your rectum.

If you are pregnant and don't want to get hemorrhoids, lie on your left side as much as possible when you're lying down. This takes the venous pressure off the anal veins and you will be much less likely to get hemorrhoids. If you already have hemorrhoids, they won't usually get bigger if you adopt that sleeping or resting position.

Summary

Hemorrhoids are a matter of too much pressure on the anal veins and the anal plexus. Pressure can come from things you can do something about, like lack of exercise, a constipating diet and straining at stool. Pressure can also come from things you can't do anything about, like a congenital lack of valves in the anal veins or liver ascites. Anything that increases the blood pressure in the anal plexus can (and usually does) lead to hemorrhoids. There are internal and external hemorrhoids and many people who have one kind of hemorrhoid also have the other. In the next chap-

ter, we'll take a look at the symptoms of hemorrhoids and how you know you have them.

Chapter 4: How Do You Know You Have Hemorrhoids?

Believe it or not, some people have hemorrhoids and don't know it. They may feel fullness in the anal area and nothing else. Others may have painless bleeding whenever they stool. The bleeding might come only when the bowel movement is particularly hard or it can happen with every stool. This is typical of internal hemorrhoids.

External hemorrhoids can itch, especially when you're not careful about cleaning the stool around the lumps. The itching represents inflammation of the hemorrhoids and can be made better by wiping with a moist towelette or simply wiping several times until the tissue comes clean. Hemorrhoids like these can be painful as well.

There is a big difference in symptoms when you have internal hemorrhoids compared to having external hemorrhoids. External hemorrhoids are painful and itch more. Blood can clot within an external hemorrhoid, resulting in a "thrombosed external hemorrhoid". This condition is extremely painful and the lump that was there tends to get bigger and harder to the touch. This type of hemorrhoid can bleed upon straining to pass a stool.

Internal hemorrhoids usually offer up bleeding as their only symptoms. The bleeding is usually bright red and will be around the stool and in the toilet bowl. If an internal hemorrhoid is big enough, it could prolapse out of the anus after stooling and might need to be manually reduced back into the rectum.

The Range of Symptoms

Hemorrhoids tend not to go from asymptomatic to severely symptomatic. They tend to go on a gradation that starts with minor irritation and goes on up to severe irritation. The progression of the disease process is like this:

- Itching usually comes first. The hemorrhoids become itchy when they get continually soiled. In addition, hemorrhoids in the early stages will seep mucus. The mucus is irritating to the skin and it creates itching.

- Skin irritation can then happen. This happens when large hemorrhoids bulge from the anus (internal hemorrhoids). They, too, secrete mucus and cause irritation of the surrounding tissue.

- Discomfort happens next. It gives you the feeling of needing to pass a stool even if you have passed a bowel movement recently. This is caused by a bulging of the hemorrhoid in the anal canal. The bigger the hemorrhoid, the greater is the discomfort experienced.

- Pain is seen more in external hemorrhoids than in internal hemorrhoids. If an internal hemorrhoid prolapses through the rectum and cannot be reduced, it can cause pain.

- Severe pain comes from a strangulated or thrombosed hemorrhoid. It tends not to get better unless there is medical treatment.

Remember that rectal bleeding and rectal pain are the exact symptoms caused by colon or anal cancer. The bleeding can be more mixed within the stool but can also be bright red blood outside the stool. If you are over 50 or have a strong family history of colon cancer should have a colonoscopy test to make sure they don't have colorectal cancer or colonic polyps.

Summary

How do you know if you have hemorrhoids? You may have painless bleeding with stools. You may have itching are an irritated feeling in the anal area. You could have discomfort or pain in the perianal area. You might be able to feel swollen lumps around the anus or you might feel no lumps unless you have a hard bowel movement. Feces can leak in some circumstances and this causes a greater itching and irritation.

Don't forget that internal hemorrhoids usually have very different symptoms from external hemorrhoids. While internal hemorrhoids bleed but don't hurt much, external hemorrhoids bleed less but are more irritating and painful. A person can have just internal hemorrhoids, just external hemorrhoids or both internal and external hemorrhoids. While both types of hemorrhoids are relatively benign, you might need to see a doctor. In the next chapter, we'll talk about when is the appropriate time to seek medical advice.

Chapter 5: Do You Need Medical Treatment?

Not everyone needs to see the doctor for their hemorrhoids. If the hemorrhoids are mild, soaking in the tub and practicing healthy bowel habits are generally enough. They make over the counter creams and preparations for hemorrhoids that work well for most people. Some of the great ways to treat hemorrhoids are listed below.

Home Treatments for Hemorrhoids

There are several great treatments for hemorrhoids. One of them is **Hem-B-Gone**. This is a product which contains horse chestnut, bilberry and ginger. These together give the product anti-inflammatory, astringent, vein strengthening and anti-swelling properties. This product scores high among other remedies because it contains only pharmaceutical extracts of the ingredients listed below. The product is safe and potent, it is recommended by many practitioners of alternative medicine for hemorrhoidal relief.

Another product is **Avatrol**. This contains some of the same ingredients, except witch hazel, but the ingredients aren't as strong as with the above product. It contains the greatest ingredient list of all hemorrhoid products. It takes about a month of continuous use for optimum results.

And then there's **ZenMed**. This is an external cream for use only in the treatment of external hemorrhoids. It contains witch hazel distillate, sage, rosemary, and rose essence, all of which soothe the itch and pain of external hemorrhoids. It cannot be used for internal hemorrhoids.

Hem-Relief is one of the oldest preparations for hemorrhoids available. It contains witch hazel and horse chestnut but little else. It doesn't contain the purified extracts of ingredients than some other products with essentially the same ingredients.

Preparation H Suppositories are used primarily for internal hemorrhoids. It contains preparations that soothe inflamed tissues and a vasoconstrictor called phenylephrine HCl that shrinks hemorrhoidal tissue. Because of the phenylephrine, it can be used for external hemorrhoids even though it is taken as a suppository.

Zinc Oxide is the same ingredient in ointments for infant diaper rash. It protects the chafing of the hemorrhoid and dries out the tissue. Some doctors simply recommend using petroleum jelly to keep the moisture off the hemorrhoid.

You can use suppositories made by **Tucks** for up to seven days when hemorrhoids flare but some of the ingredients in these suppositories are irritating to anal tissue if used too long.

Hydrocortisone 1 percent ointment is a corticosteroid medication that soothes the inflammation of hemorrhoidal tissue. It is recommended that you use these products for no longer than two weeks because they are capable of thinning the skin.

PILEX, as described in Chapter 2, has worked wonders for me personally, though it is quite expensive.

Finally, you can use products that contain a local anesthetic. It numbs the area and gives you several hours of relief. Many people are allergic to these products, however, so it pays to talk to your doctor about them or do a test on less sensitive skin.

Tips for Home Treatment

First of all you need to try and not make hemorrhoids worse. Use a cleansing agent such as **Balneal** or toilet paper moistened with a bit of water so you can gently blot the anus. Don't rub the area as that can inflame it. Allow yourself to rinse your anal area in the shower instead of using toilet paper. Pat the area dry with a soft cloth or towel. Don't use any soaps that contain a lot of perfumes or dyes. Consider installing a bidet on your toilet. It is well worth the investment for people with hemorrhoids.

Pain and swelling can be relieved through the use of acetaminophen, aspirin or other NSAIDS like naproxen and ibuprofen. For severe pain, put ice on the hemorrhoids ten minutes at a time several times a day. After the ice has been applied, follow that up by using a warm compress on the anal area for an additional 10-20 minutes.

Try a sitz bath if all else fails. You fill the tub with just enough water to cover the anus. Sit in it and let water from the tap flow on the anal area, especially after a bowel movement. Allow yourself to soak for about15 minutes. The water should be medium warm and not too hot.

In serious cases, allow yourself a day of bed rest on your left side or stomach. This takes the pressure off swollen veins and you will feel better after several hours. Don't sit for long periods of time or stand for a long time, especially when the hemorrhoids are aggravated.

Wear cotton underwear so the sweat from that area has a chance to breathe. Loose clothing helps take the pressure off the hemorrhoids and you'll feel better.

When to see the Doctor

If home remedies and common sense don't seem to help the hemorrhoidal problem, you may need to see the doctor. See your primary care doctor anytime the bleeding seems excessive. You can actually get anemic from heavily bleeding hemorrhoids.

If you have an internal hemorrhoid that won't reduce or reduces with difficulty, this may be a surgical issue that needs the help and advice of a surgeon, usually a general surgeon or a colorectal surgeon.

You'd also see a colorectal surgeon if the bleeding hasn't been thoroughly investigated yet. In that case, you'd see the surgeon after taking a preparation that cleans out the colon so you could have a colonoscopy, which is a camera study using a long tube that is snaked through the colon. Any polyps, which are pre-cursors to colon cancer, are removed and, if colon cancer appears to be present, it can be biopsied and sent to the lab for evaluation. The good news is that, if the colonoscopy is negative, you don't need another one for ten years and you can be rest assured you're dealing with just hemorrhoids.

The doctor can also prescribe stronger creams, such as hydrocortisone 2.5 percent for the inflammation if the over the counter cream fails to be effective.

Summary

Most people try home remedies to take care of their hemorrhoids. There are scores of over the counter preparations, including creams, ointments, and suppositories that ease the itching, inflammation and swelling of external and internal hemorrhoids. There are tips and tricks to keep the hemorrhoids at bay and when these fail or when symptoms become too severe, it's time to see the doctor for further evaluation and management. In the next chapter, we'll take a look at the surgical options for the management of hemorrhoids.

Chapter 6: Medical and Surgical Options for Hemorrhoids

The good news is that most people who have hemorrhoids can do something about them using home remedies or doctor's medications. Hemorrhoids are lifelong problems, however, so some people choose to have a surgical solution to their problem. There are several types of surgical options that are reserved for hemorrhoids that bleed profusely or for hemorrhoids that are so painful that they aren't treated effectively with pain medications.

Hemorrhoidectomy

The main surgery used to remove hemorrhoids is known as a hemorrhoidectomy. During this procedure, the surgeon makes cuts around the anus and actually cuts away the hemorrhoidal cushions, removing the hemorrhoids. It can be done under general anesthesia or under local anesthesia using a local numbing medication and sedation to keep the patient calm.

When the hemorrhoids are cut out, the area is stitched back together and the patient can go home after just a few hours of rest. Because cutting and stitching are involved, the anal area can be extremely tender and painful after a hemorrhoidectomy so that pain medications are given to ease the pain over the next few days.

Prolapsed Hemorrhoid Treatment

If the internal hemorrhoids slip out of the anal canal and are on the outside of the body, a PPH is performed, which stands for Procedure for Prolapse and Hemorrhoids. This is fortunately a minimally invasive procedure which can be used for prolapsed internal hemorrhoids or regular hemorrhoids.

In the procedure, a surgical stapler is used to cut off the blood supply to the hemorrhoids that eventually shrivel up and die. It takes the hemorrhoids and moves them to be higher within the anus. This is the part of the anus that has fewer pain nerve endings so they don't tend to hurt very much.

The advantages of the PPH procedure include:

- Faster recovery time
- Decreased pain
- Less itching and bleeding
- Fewer complications

Miscellaneous Treatment Options

These range from low tech options to high tech, state of the art techniques for decreasing the size of hemorrhoids:

- **Laser technique**. This uses laser to send a beam of laser energy to burn away hemorrhoids with very little bleeding and discomfort.

- **Rubber band technique**. This is a very successful low tech technique and involves a rubber band being placed around the base of the hemorrhoid. It cuts off the blood supply and eventually the tissue dies and falls off. This is a very painless procedure.

- **Sclerotherapy**. This is when a corrosive chemical solution is injected around the hemorrhoid, cutting off the blood supply to the hemorrhoid. It shrinks the hemorrhoid or causes the hemorrhoid to fall off.

The minimally invasive procedures listed above are less painful than a hemorrhoidectomy but might not have the long term benefit of a hemorrhoidectomy. See what your doctor recommends for you.

Risks of Hemorrhoid Surgery

In general, hemorrhoid surgery is extremely safe but does carry a few minor risks:

- Bleeding at the time of surgery or after surgery

- Infection, because the surgery is not being done in a particularly clean area

- Anesthesia reactions or allergies

- Problems urinating can happen because the pain of the surgery won't allow the muscles to relax, allowing the urine to flow.

- There can be fecal incontinence or the inability to control the bowels because of the muscle weakness following surgery. You can have the involuntary letting go of gas or feces.

Managing Pain after Hemorrhoid Surgery

The most common problem after hemorrhoidectomy or less invasive procedures is pain, which is made worse with bowel movements. One can take Tylenol, Advil or Anaprox to ease the pain. It is probably not a good idea to take opioid medication for pain as this can cause constipation and can make the hemorrhoidal pain worse.

You can soak in the bath tub in warm water to ease the operative pain. Stool softeners help your bowel movements go easier. If you instead strain at your stool, your hemorrhoids might come back. It generally takes a couple of weeks to fully recover from a hemorrhoidectomy but can take as long as six weeks.

Effectiveness of Hemorrhoid Surgery

Hemorrhoidal surgery is extremely effective at getting rid of the pain and itching of hemorrhoids. If you continue to practice good hemorrhoidal hygiene, your hemorrhoids should stay at bay. If you develop constipation again on a regular basis, you may get your hemorrhoids back again.

After hemorrhoid surgery, you should call the doctor if you have a great deal of bleeding, if you get a fever, if you find yourself unable to urinate or if you cannot have a bowel movement. Most people with hemorrhoidal surgery do just fine without any of the major complications.

After you have hemorrhoidal surgery, there are things you can do to keep them from coming back. You need to keep your stools very soft but not to the point of diarrhea. This means drinking plenty of fluids each day, eating a high fiber diet and getting enough exercise once you recover from the surgery. You may be a candidate for hemorrhoidal medications like Citrucel or Metamucil that will add bulk to the stool so your stools are regular and not constipated.

Summary

Surgeries are possible in the management of hemorrhoids. There is the hemorrhoidectomy, the most invasive of all hemorrhoidal surgeries. There are also less invasive procedures such as sclerotherapy, laser procedures, and rubber band procedures that act on the blood supply to hemorrhoids.

Hemorrhoid surgery is generally very safe and effective. There can be bleeding or fever after the surgery or even difficulty urinating following the procedure. The way to prevent reoccurrence of the hemorrhoids is to avoid constipation at all costs. It may mean you take a bulk laxative for a period of time after the procedure.

Chapter 7: Tips for Avoiding Hemorrhoids

If you want to avoid getting hemorrhoids in the first place or you're starting to get the symptoms of hemorrhoids and don't want to get them any further, there are things you can do to prevent hemorrhoids or at least keep them from getting any worse. In fact, the vast majority of hemorrhoid sufferers manage their symptoms at home satisfactorily.

While hemorrhoids are not generally serious, they can cause significant discomfort, especially with bowel movements, are embarrassing and often itch. For these and other reasons, you need a few tips as to how to keep your hemorrhoids under control:

- **Eat more fiber.** The hemorrhoids you are experiencing are a direct result of constipation. By eating more fiber, you can add more bulk to your diet and decrease the degree of constipation you have. You will strain less when you have a bowel movement and you will have less pressure on your hemorrhoids. Try avocados, apples, whole grains like bran and oats, spinach carrots, broccoli, bananas, grapefruits and oranges, to name a few.

If a fiber-rich diet isn't something you're used to, increase the amount of fiber in your diet gradually. Too much fiber when you're not used to it can cause gas excess, bloating and flatulence. Chapter 9 provides more tips on fighting hemorrhoids through diet. In Chapter 10 you will find a list of recipes designed for hemorrhoid patients.

- **Exercise as often as you can.** Exercise improves your muscle tone and circulation; it can prevent constipation, which leads to hemorrhoids. The idea is to do light to moderate exercise and not to overdo it. If you do strenuous exercises and weight lifting while already having hemorrhoids, you can make the hemorrhoids worse. Instead of heavy weight lifting, which can increase the pressure in the hemorrhoidal cushions, try walking, light jogging or even swimming. Yoga is a great exercise that won't make hemorrhoids worse.

- **Don't sit down or stand for a long time.** This means that you probably shouldn't have a job where you're sitting behind a computer all the time or standing behind a cash register. This puts extra pressure on the hemorrhoidal cushions and increases hemorrhoids. If you work sitting down, find things to do to get yourself out of the cubicle whenever possible. Don't read on the toilet either.

- **Stool softeners and fiber supplements are great.** These are for people that can't get enough fiber in their diet and need to take something more to ease bowel movements. Fiber supplements and stool softeners will do a lot make your stools softer and more bulky. Stool softeners are best used when they are used on a temporary basis.

- **Have comfortable bowel movements.** Make the best possible atmosphere for passing stools. Try not to feel rushed about the process and make sure you go to the restroom as soon as you feel the urge. Don't hold your breath while trying to pass stool. Try to create a regular schedule around when to have bowel movements; your body will learn to get the idea. If you hold the urge to stool, your stool will only harden and that will lead to increased hemorrhoidal pressure. If you already have hemorrhoids, blot the area with a piece of wet toilet paper or a moist towelette.

- **Drink a lot of water.** Water hydrates your stool, allowing it to be softer. The fluid should be something like water, juice or milk and not sodas or alcohol. Soda and alcohol can adversely affect bowel movements. Other liquids you shouldn't take in are green tea, coffee and other drinks high in caffeine like energy drinks. Caffeine is a diuretic that prevents water from going through the stools but rather through the urine. When you're dehydrated, you have hard stools that put pressure on the hemorrhoidal cushions. Water adds to the fiber and increases the bulk of the stool.

- **Don't lift heavy objects.** Heavy lifting can strain the veins around the rectum, causing hemorrhoids. This applies to heavy objects on the job and heavy lifting as a part of weight lifting. If you need to lift something heavy, try not to hold your breath when you lift and get assistance from others to lift an object you shouldn't be lifting yourself.

- **Sit in a sitz bath.** If you already have hemorrhoids, draw a warm bath with 6-8 inches of water in it. Add a cup of Epsom salts. Sit in the bath about 10-15 minutes. It can reduce the swelling of hemorrhoids and can soothe the feelings you're having with your hemorrhoids.

- **Use Non-prescription cream, ointment or suppositories.** There are many non-prescription ointments, creams or suppositories that soothe the irritation of hemorrhoids, both internal and external hemorrhoids. You can even use nonmedicated petroleum jelly on your sensitive hemorrhoids.

- **Use a pain relieving pad.** Put Epsom salts in a sanitary napkin and use them to cover the hemorrhoids for some relief. You can also use medicated Tucks pads, tucked into the hemorrhoids. They contain witch hazel for comfort.

Try the above home remedies as they are inexpensive and can give you the chance of having relief without having expensive surgery or misery.

Chapter 8: Herbal Remedies for Hemorrhoids

Centuries before modern medicine came up with surgeries and modern treatments, ancient herbalists used herbal remedies, many of which are still used today. In fact, since no miracle cure for hemorrhoids has yet been discovered for hemorrhoids, herbs are as good a treatment for hemorrhoids as the most modern medicine. The secret is that the modern medicines used for hemorrhoids are often based on herbs. Let's look at some excellent herbal remedies for hemorrhoids:

- **Bioflavonoids**. These are plant compounds believed to stabilize and strengthen the walls of blood vessels. They also decrease inflammation. They lessen anal pain and anal discharge, especially during an acute attack of hemorrhoids. There are few side effects and can be used in hemorrhoids related to pneumonia. The bioflavonoid derived from tangeretin shouldn't be used by those taking tamoxifen for the treatment of breast cancer.

Citrus fruits are high in flavonoids such as diosmin, oxerutins, and herperidin and are particularly helpful in the management of hemorrhoids. There is a product called Daflon that is made with citrus bioflavonoids. It is known to improve hemorrhoidal symptoms among pregnant women who take it for at least four days. The pain, bleeding, itching, discharge and heavy sensation are markedly minimized.

- **Apple cider vinegar, cayenne and honey.** This is mixed with hot water and is sipped before meals and during meals. It is supposed to protect your capillaries against toxic damage as well as protecting digestion. Try a cup of vinegar, a cup of honey and 2-4 cups of distilled hot water. Add 1/4 teaspoon of cayenne pepper (you can use more as your body gets used to it). Mix and refrigerate, consuming cupfuls with meals until it clears up the problem. It can be drunk cold if you like it that way better.

- **Witch Hazel.** This is a product that comes in many forms, including creams, liquids and compresses. It is created from the bark of a plant called Hamamelis virginiana. It is only an external product and is applied directly to the anal and perianal area. It is known to decrease the bleeding caused by hemorrhoids and is an astringent, drying up the tissue. It can also relieve the symptoms of pain, swelling and itching seen in hemorrhoids.

- **Butcher's Broom.** This is also known as the plant Ruscus aculeatus. Other names include box holly, knee holly and sweet broom. It was once used by European butchers to clean their chopping blocks. It has been used for hundreds of years to treat hemorrhoids and improve the poor circulation sometimes seen in varicose veins. Butcher's broom extract is anti-inflammatory and constricts swollen veins by improving the tone and integrity of veins, shrinking hemorrhoidal tissue. It has an active compound, known as ruscogen.

Butcher's broom can be taken in tea form or capsule form. The tea tastes a bit bitter so you should add some honey or stevia to make it sweeter. Steep a teaspoon of butcher's broom in a cup of hot water for ten to 15 minutes. There are products of butcher's broom that come in compresses or ointments.

It can't be taken, especially internally, by those who have high blood pressure, are pregnant, are nursing or who have BPH (benign prostatic hypertrophy). People taking MAO inhibitors or alpha blockers shouldn't take butcher's broom.

- **Horse Chestnut.** This comes from the herb called Aesculus hippocastanum is similar to butcher's broom because it works when the circulation around the anus is poor. It relieves itching, swelling and inflammation of hemorrhoids and strengthens the blood vessel walls. It has an active compound called aescin.

Horse chestnut is taken in tea or capsule form. Compresses can be made for external application. It shouldn't be taken if you have an allergy to horse chestnut or if you have a bleeding disorder or are taking blood thinners. Horse chestnut should be made only out of the seeds, young branches or bark of the plant because the other parts of the plant are considered poisonous. Rare side effects of horse chestnut include bleeding complications, bruising, liver damage or kidney damage.

- **Triphala**. This is a compound belonging to Ayurvedic medicine. It is a compound made from three separate fruits and it acts as a bowel tonic, decreasing constipation without being too harsh on the bowels.

- **White Oak Bark and Comfrey Root.** These are ground to a powder and mixed with cocoa butter to make a suppository. Insert one refrigerated suppository in the rectum each night before going to bed. The herbs strengthen the tissue so that you don't have hemorrhoids so big. It is intended to be done several nights in a row until the hemorrhoids are healed.

- **Stone root.** This is an herbal remedy that strengthens hemorrhoidal tissue. It is taken one teaspoon at a time mixed with one cup of water and taken twice a day, half a cup per time.

- **Marshmallow root, chamomile flowers and flaxseed**. These are mixed as a tea and are used to soften the bowel and ease the pressure on the hemorrhoids.

- **For hard stools:** try a half cup of aloe juice twice daily or use tonics containing yellow dock root or cascara bark. These are intended to be used for short periods of time and not for the long haul.

- **Witch hazel leaf and wild yam root.** One teaspoon of each herb is used in two cups of water, steeped for 20 minutes. Then add 1/2 cup aloe juice, drinking a cup of the mixture two to three times per day before meals.

Summary

Herbal remedies and hemorrhoids go hand in hand because they have centuries of experience and success in calming the pain and inflammation that comes when hemorrhoids are severe. Interestingly, the ingredients of the preparations you'll find from the pharmacy often contain the very herbal remedies you can make yourself after a trip to the herbalist or health food store.

While herbal remedies are generally safe to take, some have contraindications—situations in which taking the herbal remedy would not be considered safe. Herbal remedies taken internally are more likely to interact with other diseases or medications you are taking so make sure you talk to an herbalist, pharmacist or physician before taking one of these remedies.

Chapter 9: Eliminate Hemorrhoids through Diet

You don't have to undergo painful hemorrhoid surgery in order to have relief from this annoying and painful problem. Your diet should be a big part of how you go about fighting the pain and inflammation of hemorrhoids. There are things you should eat often ad things you should avoid. We'll take a look at both.

- **Increase your fiber intake.** Fiber is the part of plants that cannot be digested. They stay in the intestinal tract and provide bulk and an easier time of having a bowel movement. Soluble fiber like oats makes for a softer stool that is easier to pass. You will have less constipation and there will be less pressure on the hemorrhoids. Good sources of soluble fiber include flaxseed, oats, peas, beans, carrots, apples, berries, barley and psyllium. You can have psyllium as a supplement from the pharmacy as well. There is also insoluble fiber that adds bulkiness to the stool.

- **Bioflavonoids or flavonoids.** These are naturally occurring substances in plants and are the part of brightly colored fruits and vegetables that make them so colorful. Scientists have found a connection between the intake of flavonoids and improvements in the bleeding, itching and other symptoms of hemorrhoids. They are believed to strengthen blood vessels and to reduce free radical stress inside the blood vessels.

- **Eat blueberries.** Blueberries are rich in anthocyanins and therefore are good when it comes to repairing damaged proteins in the wall of blood vessels so the vascular system is improved. In addition, blueberries are high in insoluble fiber and soluble fiber in the form of pectin. If you can find wild blueberries, you can get an extra source of vitamin E as well.

- **Eat figs.** Figs have a longstanding reputation for curing constipation. Most of the fiber is in the skin of figs so eat them with the skins on. Look for figs at the grocery store or farmer's market that are plump, soft to the touch but not too mushy. They should smell sweet and mildly fresh. Figs are highly perishable so you have to buy them to last only a couple of days. You can also use dried figs for constipation. They have a shelf life of more than a year.

- **Spinach.** This is a great vegetable for those who have any intestinal tract problem, including hemorrhoids. It cleanses and regenerates the GI tract and contains Magnesium, which is necessary for proper bowel movements. Western countries have a high rate of slight magnesium deficiency and suffer constipation as a result. There isn't much magnesium in the processed foods we eat.

- **Eat Okra.** Okra is a plant native to the Western part of Africa and helps maintain an excellent gastrointestinal system. Okra contains fiber that absorbs water and adds bulk to your stool. It moves stool through the bowels, preventing constipation. Okra contains mucilage that facilitates the painful elimination of waste. Buy okra that is longer than four inches; eat them steamed or boiled. Cook it as little as possible so that it retains its healthiest nutrients and enzymes. You can even add thin slices of the vegetable to a bowel of salad greens.

- **Try beets.** Beets not only prevent constipation but they seem to prevent colon cancer as well. Beets are a high fiber vegetable so it bulks the stool. You can even eat the leafy tops of beets as these are high in fiber and in nutrients. The nutrient that makes beets red is called betacyanin, which is a phytochemical that has been shown to help fight colon cancer. Beets are truly a superfood that is great for getting rid of hemorrhoids.

- **Papaya.** This fruit can be found in just about any tropical country. It contains a lot of nutrients, include papain, which is the active ingredient in the fruit that controls constipation. Green papaya contains more papain than ripe papain. You can find unripe papain in Asian food stores.

- **Oatmeal.** Try a bowlful of oatmeal every morning. Oats are a great source of soluble fiber. It forms a gel when mixed with water; this combines with the insoluble fiber in oats for a double play of power against constipation. It is known to make stool softer and bulkier. If eating regular oats, you should soak them for a couple of hours to get rid of the phytic acid that blocks magnesium absorption in the small intestines.

- **Eat prunes.** Prunes are an excellent source of fiber and are well known to counteract constipation. Prunes contain colonic stimulants that further help you evacuate your bowels. Most of the contents of prunes stay in the bowels and add to the bulk of our stool.

- **Try Barley.** Barley contains dietary fiber that softens stool, increases stool bulk and lessens the transit time it takes for your stool to pass through the colon. The fiber in barley feeds the good bacteria in the large colon.

- **Drink plenty of water.** Water adds to stool to make the stool softer. If you don't have enough water in your diet, your stools will harden. Try to get between 6 and 10 glasses of actual water per day for the softest stools that will pass easily.

There are **foods you should avoid** if you have hemorrhoids. These are things that can cause constipation or that make you strain when you have a bowel movement and include low fiber sweets, cheese, meat, fizzy drinks, alcohol and coffee. Try to avoid spicy foods, pastries, pasta made with white flour, white bread and processed foods with a lot of sodium in them. Avoid cakes, cookies, breakfast cereals containing sugar and foods that are high in fat. Caffeine is a stimulant laxative which is not the way you want to have your bowel movements. Alcohol dehydrates the body and makes stool harder. Foods like nuts, mustard, and red pepper will contribute to having bleeding hemorrhoids. They also pass through the colon partially digested which aggravates hemorrhoids.

Summary

Pay attention to the foods you should eat when you have hemorrhoids and avoid the foods you shouldn't eat. Try to make up recipes that incorporate your need for hemorrhoid-healthy foods and keep a list of them so, when you go to the store, you can have the recipes handy. To help you out, the next chapter is a list of recipes for dishes you can make that are healthy for your hemorrhoids.

Chapter 10: Hemorrhoid-Free Recipes

Here are some fantastic recipes that can keep hemorrhoids at bay and can help your diet stay as healthy as possible:

Avocado, Tomato and Arugula Salad

This provides a great deal of fiber and has bioflavonoids for good colon health.

Ingredients:
- 2 c halved cherry tomatoes
- 3 c small arugula leaves
- 2 tbsp olive oil
- 1/4 c sun-dried tomatoes, chopped up
- 1 tbsp balsamic vinegar
- 2 small, peeled and pitted avocadoes, sliced

Directions:

Using a plastic bowl, toss cherry tomatoes, arugula, sun-dried tomatoes, olive oil and vinegar. Put onto plates, serving each plate with a few slices of avocado.

Carrot and Beet Ginger Salad

Both beets and carrots are high in fiber so as to prevent constipation and hemorrhoidal inflammation. Betacyanin is found in beets; it is a phytochemical that also fights colon cancer.

Ingredients:

- 1/2 c grated organic carrots
- 1/2 c grated raw beets
- 2 tbsp olive oil
- 1/2 tsp minced fresh ginger
- 1/8 tsp salt

Directions:

Mix grated vegetables in a little bowl. Combine the rest of the ingredients in a separate bowl and drizzle the dressing over the carrot and beet salad. Toss this salad well and enjoy.

Apple Onion Soup

Apples have the fiber you need to keep hemorrhoids away. The entire recipes promote regular bowel movements so the chances of having inflamed hemorrhoids are less.

Ingredients:

- 1 tbsp canola oil
- 2 sliced yellow onions
- 1 leek, chopped
- 1/2 tbsp chopped fresh rosemary
- 1/2 tbsp chopped fresh thyme
- 3 apples, diced and cored
- 6 c low sodium veggie broth

Directions:

Heat canola oil in medium pan until hot. Sauté the onions until golden brown. Add broth and boil over medium heat. Add the apples and set to simmer on medium-low. Simmer apples until tender—about ten minutes.

Avocado and Carrot Salad

These vegetables both have a lot of fiber that can bulk the stool and make bowel movements easier to have.

Ingredients:

- 4 carrots, grated and peeled
- 1 big avocado, peeled and diced
- Splash of balsamic vinegar
- Sunflower seeds, enough to taste
- Salt and pepper to taste

Directions:

Mix vegetables together in a medium bowl. Sprinkle with the remaining ingredients to your taste and cover, refrigerating for at least twenty minutes before eating.

Barley Soup

There is a lot of dietary fiber in this recipe that can increase the bulk of the stool and can shorten the time between eating and elimination of the food. Barley acts as a healthy prebiotic, feeding the healthy bacteria of the bowels. The carrots add extra fiber.

Ingredients:

- 1/3 c pearled barley
- 2/3 c water
- 1/2 c chopped onion
- 2 tbsp olive oil
- 1 c chopped carrots
- 1 2/3 c plain yogurt with active cultures of probiotics
- 2/3 c minced fresh parsley
- 2 c vegetable stock
- Salt and pepper to taste

Directions:

Boil water in a large soup pot. Simmer barley for up to 30 minutes over low heat. When water has evaporated, set aside. In a stock pot, sauté onion for 5 minutes in oil. Add vegetable stock and carrots, allow to boil. Reduce stock to a simmer and cook for twenty minutes. Add barley and let simmer for a minute or two. Take off heat and stir in yoghurt and seasonings. Serve right away.

Carrot and Beet Soup

This contains fiber that can prevent hemorrhoids. Beets contain cancer-fighting flavonoids. Your bowel movements will be healthier with this soup in your recipe collection.

Ingredients:

- 3 medium beets, diced
- 1 c chopped onions
- 1 lb carrots, diced
- 1 tbsp canola oil
- 1 tbsp fresh ginger, minced
- 6 c vegetable stock
- 2 cloves minced garlic

Directions:

Saute onion in oil until golden. Add garlic and ginger and cook for two minutes until soft. Add beets, stock and carrots. Boil first and then simmer, covered, until vegetables are tender. It should take about 25 minutes.

Asparagus with Walnuts and Quince Jam

Asparagus is very good for you and contains a lot of fiber. It is especially effective and getting rid of constipation and ridding hemorrhoids. Walnuts are also a folk remedy for constipation.

Ingredients:

- 2 lbs trimmed asparagus spears
- 2 tbsp quince jam
- 2 tsp grated fresh ginger
- 2 tbsp olive oil
- 3 tbsp walnuts
- 1 tsp lemon juice
- Salt and pepper to taste

Directions:

Steam asparagus with steamer until it is slightly tender and slightly crisp, about 3-5 minutes. Put asparagus on a serving plate. Whisk together quince jam, ginger, olive oil, lemon juice, pepper and salt. Pour this over the asparagus and top with chopped walnuts.

Pasta with Nettle Pesto

This uses whole wheat pasta so you can make us of the pasta. Young, blanched nettle leaves won't sting you and will provide you with flavonoids to strengthen blood vessels. It is a great dish for those who have hemorrhoids.

Ingredients:

- 2 c blanched young nettle leaves
- 1/3 c chopped walnuts
- 4 cloves peeled garlic
- 1/3 c grated Parmesan cheese
- 1/3 c olive oil
- 12 ounces whole wheat pasta

Directions:

Mix garlic, nettle leaves, and walnuts inside a food processor, adding olive oil until smooth. Stir in Parmesan cheese and cook pasta until al dente. Drain the pasta and put it back in the pot it was cooked in. Add pesto and toss. Place on serving plates.

Barley and Broccoli Soup

Both of these ingredients are rich in dietary fiber so your stools will be soft and will have a shorter transit time through the GI tract. Barley has prebiotics so your healthy bacteria will be properly fed. The bacteria then produce butyric acid, which is healthy for your colon.

Ingredients:

- 1 carrot, diced
- 1/4 c chopped onion
- 1 stalk finely chopped celery
- 4 c broccoli florets
- 1 tbsp olive oil
- 5 c vegetable broth
- 1/2 c cooked pearled broccoli
- 1 can stewed tomatoes
- 4 cloves minced garlic
- 1 tsp thyme
- 1/4 tsp dried marjoram
- Salt and pepper to taste

Directions:

Cook onion in olive oil in stock pot for 4-5 minutes or until onions are soft and translucent. Add vegetable broth and boil. Reduce to a simmer and add veggies to broth, simmering until veggies are tender. Add barley, canned tomatoes, marjoram, thyme, garlic and salt/pepper. Simmer for two minutes until heated through.

Asparagus, Stir-Fried with Quinoa Noodles

This is a delicious asparagus dish that also fights hemorrhoids. Asparagus contains inulin, which is a special type of fiber that prevents constipation.

Ingredients:

- 1 tbsp olive oil
- 2 bundles of asparagus, cut into bite sized pieces
- 3 tsp minced fresh ginger
- 2 slivered garlic cloves
- 1/2 tbsp sugar
- 1 tbsp soy sauce
- 12 ounces dried quinoa noodles
- 3.5 tbsp vegetable stock

Directions:

Use wok and stir fry garlic and ginger for a minute or two. Add asparagus and heat. In a small bowl, mix sugar, soy sauce, and stock, pouring over asparagus. Simmer mixture until asparagus is tender, which should take 3-5 minutes. Cook noodles until al dente and mix with vegetable mixture.

Spinach Soup with Boiled Eggs

This Scandinavian dish has bioflavonoids for hemorrhoid health. Spinach is good for the whole GI tract and cleanses/regenerates the GI tract.

Ingredients:

- 10 ounces fresh spinach leaves
- 2 tbsp olive oil
- 2 c water
- 2 c organic milk
- 1 chopped onion, yellow
- 3 tbsp flour
- Salt to taste
- Nutmeg to taste
- White pepper to taste
- 4 halved boiled eggs

Directions:

Wash and chop spinach into coarse chunks. Saute onion in olive oil until onions are golden brown. Add water and spinach. Bring to a boil and cook until spinach is wilted. Blend with a hand mixer until mixture is smooth. Whisk together cold milk and flour and pour into saucepan, allowing it to whisk with spinach mixture. Allow to boil and then simmer until thickened. Season with salt, nutmeg and pepper. Pour into serving dishes and garnish with halves of eggs.

Bean and Barley Soup

This contains a great deal of dietary fiber that softens the stool and prevents constipation. Barley also contains prebiotics that feed healthy colonic bacteria for overall good colon health.

Ingredients:

- 1 diced carrot
- 1/4 c chopped onion
- 1 stalk celery, chopped finely
- 1 tbsp olive oil
- 5 c vegetable broth
- 1/2 c cooked white beans
- 1/2 c cooked pearled barley
- 1/4 c canned tomatoes
- 4 cloves minced garlic
- 3 tbsp chopped fresh basil
- 1/2 tsp dried rosemary
- Salt and pepper to taste

Directions:

Take a soup pot and sauté onion in oil for 4-5 minute. Add celery and carrots, simmering for about 3 minutes. Add broth and boil, then simmer for several minutes until carrots and celery are soft. Add cooked barley, beans, tomatoes, garlic and spices. Simmer for two minutes. Season with salt and pepper before serving warm.

Nettle Soup

Nettle contains nutrients that help to keep blood vessels strong and elastic. This is a perfect soup for the prevention of hemorrhoids.

Ingredients:

- 4 ounces fresh spinach leaves
- 6 ounces young nettle tips
- 2 tablespoons olive oil
- 2 chopped shallots
- 3 c skim milk
- 2 c water
- 3 tbsp flour
- White pepper to taste
- Nutmeg to taste
- Salt to taste
- Yogurt with active cultures for a garnish

Directions:

Wash vegetables and chop coarsely. Saute onion in olive oil until golden brown.

Add water spinach and nettle, cooking to a boil until nettle and spinach are wilted. Blend with hand blender until you have a smooth mixture. Whisk in cold milk and flour into a small bowl. Whisk into soup mixture and boil until thickened. Add spices and remove from heat. Pour into bowls and garnish with swirled yogurt.

Winter Pea Soup

Peas are loaded with healthful fiber so they help those who are prone to hemorrhoidal irritation. The watercress leaves add spice to this great soup.

Ingredients:

- 1 large potato
- 30 ounces of frozen peas
- 3 ounces of watercress
- 1 large chopped onion
- 1 crushed clove garlic
- 6 c chicken or vegetable stock
- Dash salt & pepper

Directions:

Leave crushed garlic aside for at least 5-10 minutes. This will maximize garlic's health benefits. Meanwhile, chop onion and peel & dice potato. Add 3 tbsp of chicken stock to onion and garlic. Add potatoes and rest of stock. Boil this and let simmer until potato is cooked (about 15 minutes). Add peas and simmer for 3 minutes. Simmer with watercress until everything is soft, about 1 minute. Let cool a bit. Blend with a handheld blender until smooth. Add salt & pepper to taste.

Smoked Salmon Salad

Fish is an excellent source of protein and doesn't cause constipation. The romaine lettuce and carrots in the salad provide a good source of dietary fiber that can help you manage constipation and hemorrhoids.

Ingredients:

- 5 oz thinly sliced smoked salmon
- 1 small head of romaine lettuce
- 2 diced tomatoes
- 4 sliced radishes
- 1/2 cucumber, peeled and diced
- 1 carrot, sliced diagonally
- Juice from half a lemon
- 1 tsp minced ginger root
- 1 tbsp canola oil

Directions:

Set romaine lettuce in an arrangement on two plates. Add salmon, carrots, tomatoes, radishes and cucumber. Take lemon juice, canola oil and ginger, shaking them in a jar. Pour this dressing over the lettuce and salmon mixture. Eat heartily.

Blueberry Muesli

Blueberries are some of the best foods to eat. They are high in fiber and also help repair damaged areas of blood vessel walls. They promote the health of the entire vascular system and contain a large amount of vitamin E.

Ingredients:

- 1.5 c rolled oats
- 1/2 c chopped dried apples
- 1/2 c chopped walnuts
- 2 tsp ground cinnamon
- 2 c wild blueberries
- 3 tbsp brown sugar
- Apple juice for serving

Directions:

Preheat oven to 325 degrees F. Mix together the oats, sugar and cinnamon in a bowl and spread the combination on a nonstick baking pan. Toast for about 10 minutes, stirring occasionally. Be careful not to burn it. Remove mixture from oven and allow to cool. Pour into a larger bowl with apples and walnuts. Put mixture in bowls and add blueberries. Serve along with apple juice.

Whole Wheat Muffins with Bananas

These flavorful muffins have the fiber to prevent hemorrhoids. Bananas, too, have fructo-oligosaccharides or FOS that help digestion problems like constipation. Walnuts in the muffins take care of constipation.

Ingredients:

- 1/3 c brown sugar
- 1 c whole wheat flour
- 2/3 c chopped walnuts
- 1/2 tsp baking powder
- 1/4 tsp salt
- 2 medium sliced bananas
- 1/4 c almond milk
- 1 lightly beaten egg

Directions:

Set oven to 350 degrees F/ Mix dry ingredients into a bowl and in a separate bowl, mash the bananas using a fork. Add almond milk and egg to bananas and the mix the dry ingredients with the wet ingredients. Put batter into muffin tins with papers or use nonstick tins. Bake in oven for 30-40 minutes and send to cooling rack.

Carrot Muffins

Carrots are an excellent source of vegetable fiber. The muffins also contain guar gum and flaxseed that fight hemorrhoids and constipation.

Ingredients:

- 1 c rice milk
- 1 egg
- 2 c gluten-free flour
- 4 tbsp canola oil
- 1 tsp guar gum
- 1 tbsp flaxseed meal
- 3.5 tsp baking powder
- 1/2 tsp salt
- 1/4 c brown sugar
- 1 tsp cinnamon
- 1 c grated carrots
- 1/4 c raisins

Directions:

Set oven to 400 degrees F. Beat wet ingredients together and put dry ingredients together in a different bowl. Mix dry and wet ingredients together. Fold in the raisins and carrots. Use paper cups to fill muffins and bake for 20 minutes.

Muesli with Grapes and Pears

This muesli will get your bowels going smoothly with lots of soluble fiber that will bulk up the stool. It contains pears that contain sorbitol, a familiar laxative that draws water into the colon.

Ingredients:

- 1/2 c puffed buckwheat
- 1.5 c rolled oats
- 2 tsp cinnamon
- 1/2 c dried chopped apples
- 2 c diced pears
- 1 c halved red grapes
- 3 tbsp brown sugar
- Rice milk for serving

Directions:

Set oven to 325 degrees F. Spread oats on baking tray and toast for about 10 minutes. Be careful that they don't burn. Let them cool and then put them in a glass bowl and add water. Soak overnight in refrigerator. Add puffed buckwheat, apples, brown sugar and cinnamon to oats. Stir well. Divide into bowls and top with grapes and pears. Serve with the rice milk.

Muesli with Apples

This mixture of cereal will get your bowels going with plenty of healthy fiber and pectin, reducing the risk of inflamed and tender hemorrhoids.

Ingredients:

- 1.5 cups toasted rolled oats
- 1/2 c wheat germ
- 1.5 c diced apples
- 2 tsp cinnamon
- 2 tbsp brown sugar
- Organic yogurt with active probiotic cultures

Directions:

Set oven to 325 degrees F. Mix oats, cinnamon and brown sugar in a bowl and toast for ten minutes on a nonstick baking sheet. Remove from oven and cool. Put mixture in large bowl and stir together with wheat germ. Put in two serving bowls and top with apples and raspberries. Serve together with yogurt.

First Class Fiber Muffins

This muffin recipe supplies you with the fiber you need to have easy bowel movements. It's positively loaded with fiber!

Ingredients:

- 1 c nonfat milk
- 1.5 c wheat bran
- 1/2 c applesauce
- 1 egg
- 1/2 c regular flour
- 1/2 c whole wheat flour
- 2/3 c brown sugar
- 1 tsp baking powder
- 1 tsp baking soda
- 1/2 tsp salt
- 1 c organic chopped apples

Directions:

Set oven to 375 degrees F. Mix milk and wheat bran, letting it sit for 15 minutes. Whisk applesauce, brown sugar and egg in separate bowl and stir in bran mixture. In a smaller bowl, mix all the dry ingredients together and then mix wet and dry ingredients together until just mixed together. Fill muffin cups about two thirds full with batter and bake for 15-20 minutes.

Bircher Muesli

This is the original muesli invented by the Swiss doctor Maximilian Bircher-Brenner in the late 1800s. It was recommended to patients who had digestive problems and constipation.

Ingredients:

- 1 tbsp rolled oats
- 3 tsp water
- 1 tbsp sweetened condensed milk
- 2 tsp lemon juice
- 2 apples diced with skins
- 1 tbsp ground almonds

Directions:

Mix oats with water and allow to refrigerate overnight. This breaks down the enzymes in the oats that then neutralize the phytic acid in the oats. Phytic acid can impair nutrient absorption. Dice or grate apples and add them to milk and lemon juice. Mix with oats. Sprinkle with ground almonds and eat heartily.

Conclusion

Hemorrhoids are extremely common. It is estimated that half of all Americans will struggle with hemorrhoids but only a fraction of these people will seek medical attention for their problem. Hemorrhoids are basically swollen, varicose veins of the hemorrhoidal veins. In reality, it isn't the veins but the sinusoids, similar to veins, which get enlarged and irritated by things like constipation, having to be on your feet for a long period of time, straining at the stool and heredity.

The main symptoms of hemorrhoids are swollen lumps around the anus, rectal bleeding, itching, and pain in the anal area. There are also internal hemorrhoids that can pass through the anal canal and can get entrapped. They can go back up on their own or may need to be manually placed back into the internal aspect of the anus. In addition, hemorrhoids can get a blood clot in them, causing a thrombosed hemorrhoid: a painful hard lump that needs to be drained surgically.

Patients can seek surgical attention for their hemorrhoids. They can have a full hemorrhoidectomy or removal of the hemorrhoidal cushions. They can have laser surgery to the hemorrhoids or electrocautery to the hemorrhoids or rubber band treatment to the hemorrhoids, that later die and fall off. These surgeries are painful but you get resolution of your hemorrhoids within 3-4 weeks.

There are also many home remedies and herbal remedies for hemorrhoids. Herbal remedies often contain the same medicine in it that modern preparations for hemorrhoids have. Witch hazel and horse chestnut are popular remedies for the treatment of hemorrhoids.

Hemorrhoids can be treated with diet. Anything in the diet that reduces constipation and softens stool can reduce the chances of hemorrhoids or hemorrhoidal irritation. There are also foods that contain things that strengthen the blood vessel wall. The chapter before this gives you great recipe ideas that can help you get the most out of your diet when it comes to treating hemorrhoids.

Hemorrhoids don't have to be an annoying and irritating. There are plenty of things you can do to prevent hemorrhoids and just as many things you can do to keep your existing hemorrhoids as comfortable as possible.